KU-488-419

HOMŒOPATHY FOR THE FIRST-AIDER

By the same author
A PHYSICIAN'S POSY
THE MAGIC OF THE MINIMUM DOSE
MORE MAGIC OF THE MINIMUM DOSE
HOMOEOPATHY IN EPIDEMIC DISEASES

HOMŒOPATHY FOR THE FIRST-AIDER

by

Dr DOROTHY SHEPHERD

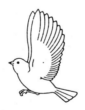

THE C. W. DANIEL COMPANY LIMITED
1 Church Path, Saffron Walden, Essex, England

First published 1945
Second (revised) Edition 1953
Second Impression May 1972
Third Impression November 1974
Fourth Impression 1977
Fifth Impression 1980
Sixth Impression 1982
Seventh Impression 1986
Eighth Impression 1989

© MRS. G.E. ROBINSON 1953

This book is sold subject to the condition that it shall not, by way of trade or otherwise, be lent, re-sold, hired out, or otherwise circulated without the publisher's prior consent in any form of binding or cover other than that in which it is published and without a similar condition including this condition being imposed on the subsequent purchaser.

ISBN 0 85032 091 7

Printed and bound in Great Britain
by Whitstable Litho Limited, Whitstable,
Kent

CONTENTS

NEW METHODS IN FIRST AID

IS there anything new under the sun? I have no desire whatsoever to underrate the old methods of first aid which have been so concisely worked out and represented in the excellent little manuals of the different Red Cross Societies and the St. John Ambulance Association. But there is a spirit of change in the air ; a new order is being freely discussed, and new methods should be welcome.

The mechanical and surgical methods of first aid have been well taught ; yet there is an absence of teaching and, if I may say so, a widespread ignorance of medicinal treatment in the first aid manuals, except for the almost universal rule of giving Aspirin for pain and hypodermic injections of Morphia for excruciating pain and shock, a procedure I deprecate thoroughly as it often leads to a craving for these drugs. For years I followed obediently the recognized, well-trodden paths of antiseptic and aseptic wound treatment, with little or no medicinal aid, other than those already mentioned. I had opportunity to study and apply first-aid methods in surgical outpatients, private practice and a munition factory in the First World War and later a minor ailment clinic. For some years now I have given up entirely the old methods and with the help of a devoted staff I have applied these comparatively new ideas which have proved not only successful, but even superior to the old ones. This must be my reason, if apologies are needed, for making known these methods in the hope that other medical practitioners and first aid personnel may be inspired to follow the lead given here to try out different lines of treatment.

I suggest that every household, school, factory and all first-aid posts should be stocked with the lotions and medicines described, so as to prevent a simple emergency from becoming a serious casualty, an essential factor in these days of easy accidents, falls and injuries on our crowded roads.

Every accident, whether minor or major, is accompanied by

shock. Though the ordinary rules for treatment of shock should be obeyed, such as applying warmth to the patient, plenty of warm blankets and hot-water bottles well wrapped up, so as to prevent accidental burns of the unconscious patient ; by far the best and most rapid improvement I have repeatedly found, follows the internal administration of *Arnica* in small and repeated doses.

ARNICA

Arnica has been known for many years all over the globe in mountainous districts, where severe falls are common, and the local peasantry in countries so far apart as Switzerland, the Tyrol and the Andes mountains in South America search diligently in the summer on the slopes and in peaty meadows for the Fall herb or *Arnica* which they dry and store up carefully for use in emergencies. We should do well not to despise the herbal lore of the countryside. *Arnica* is a treasure indeed. It does well in all injuries of the " soft parts," the muscles ; in bruises, contusions, extravasations of blood, in sprains and in strains of the muscles due to over-exertion ; whether due to tiredness after a long day of unaccustomed scrambling in mountainous country or too long a tramp after a week of sedentary work, and even the housewife when exhausted after hours of spring-cleaning will feel refreshed and will not have any tired aching limbs, if she would take a dose or two of *Arnica* when her labours are over.

Aching of the muscles and weariness after a sleepless night will disappear if *Arnica* is taken internally ; it is better than a sleeping draught and will not leave any bad effects or lead to a dangerous craving for more potent stimulants.

PAIN, ACHING, BRUISING

PAIN, due to mental and/or physical shock is relieved rapidly by *Arnica*, such as pain and swelling after a troublesome dental extraction; sprains of joints; fractured bones; even in concussions good results follow the internal administration of *Arnica*. If the patient is unconscious a small dose of *Arnica* in pilules or granules placed on the tongue will expedite the return to consciousness.

(1) A badly concussed old man with an extensively lacerated scalp wound was seen some years ago. Six stitches were put in after the scalp had been thoroughly cleansed, the patient remaining so deeply unconscious during the whole procedure that the pupil did not respond to light. Then one dose of *Arnica* was given dry on the tongue, and before I had finished sterilizing the instruments the man roused and enquired where he was. It was almost as if he had been anæsthetized, and the effect of the anæsthetic had worn off. The *Arnica* was repeated 4 hourly and within 12 hours he ate a good meal and never looked back.

(2) An elderly lady slipped on the road on a frosty day and the olecranon process of the ulna at the elbow joint was broken in three pieces. Seen within an hour of the accident, a light superficial soap and water massage removed the extravasation of the mixture of blood and serum over the elbow ; she was then X-rayed. *Arnica* had been given straight away and was repeated hourly at first and then 4 hourly, later she took it whenever she felt a return of the pain. The arm was put into a light sling, infra-red and ultra-violet light treatment and gentle massage with passive movements was given daily and the patient encouraged to flex, extend and rotate the arm gently. The result was a perfect union of the bony fragments in three weeks ; and almost 100 per cent. free movement at the elbow joint was achieved without any operation, which is a good result, especially if you consider that she was a feeble, shrivelled-up lady well

over sixty years of age with little vitality. There was never any rise of temperature or an accelerated pulse to the great astonishment of the surgeon who was called in to give a second opinion. The patient never lost any sleep, for whenever the slightest twinge of pain came along, she took a dose of *Arnica* which immediately relieved her.

Arnica tincture at the rate of one teaspoon to the pint of water or 3 to 5 drops per ounce, applied externally, relieves contusions and swelling of the soft parts, provided that there is no abrasion of the skin or any raw area ; if you do use it in such a case, erysipelas will inevitably follow from the absorption of the *Arnica*. In a case with broken skin, *Calendula tincture*, diluted 1 in 10, will replace the *Arnica* and do the work better than any antiseptic, such as Iodine and the rest, including the modern panacea, Penicillin.

A boy, ten years old, was brought into the clinic ten days after an accident due to a large brick falling on his right foot, which besides lacerating the skin broke two of the metatarsal bones. He was in hospital for over a week, then discharged as an ambulant case, still unable to walk or put his foot to the ground. When he was brought to the clinic in an invalid chair the day after his return home the Elastoplast dressing was removed at the surgery, exposing a raw suppurating wound under it. This was cleansed with warm water containing a few drops of *Calendula* and a gauze dressing moistened with *Calendula* (dilution 1–10) was applied. *Arnica* was given three times daily. The next day the boy was able to put his foot to the ground and two days later he was walking. The swelling had gone and the wound healed up rapidly, within a week he was discharged well, with a sound foot.

An old lady was found unconscious by her daughter one morning as a result of a stroke, due to cerebral hæmorrhage. *Arnica*, 4 hourly, was given for several days and within 24 hours after the first dose she became conscious and recovered completely from her hæmorrhage in a few days, regaining the use of all her limbs within ten days.

Arnica given 3 to 4 hourly after abdominal operations or after a confinement, after setting a fracture or reducing a dislocation, etc., removes pain, relieves the shock, and the patients recover much more rapidly than under Morphia. It is advisable to take *Arnica* (three doses in 24 hours) before going to a dentist to prevent shock and pain after an extraction. Hæmorrhage is frequently much lessened by such preventive measures.

It has been found that *Arnica* given internally works wonderfully well in cases of blasts from bombs, and earache due to rupture of the eardrums from the effects of blasts ; injuries to eyes from whatever causes, knocks, stones, pieces of grit in the eye are all quickly healed. Extensive bruising of face after boxing disappears within a few hours. Even blindness and cataract following on injuries to the eyes due to the throwing of stones can be prevented with 3 to 4 hourly doses of *Arnica* given for at least a week.

Our young hopefuls in imitation of their soldier brothers have pitched battles, their missiles being brickbats and stones from the debris of the ruined houses in the neighbourhood. Irreparable damage has been done to eyes many times, which either had to be removed at the hospital or traumatic cataract developed in the injured organ within a few months. At the Dispensary we have treated many severe injuries where eyebrows were laid open and the stones had glanced off the temple near the eye. With *Arnica* two or three times daily for two or three days and a local *Calendula* dressing covering the eyes, these injuries recovered within a few days and we have had no cases of traumatic cataract develop among the great number we have dealt with, far too many to describe.

A lad of twelve, while riding on a high milk delivery cart, was pitched off and fell on his face, on the stone pavement. He had just time to whisper " take me to the Sister of the Mission, not to hospital " before he lost his senses. He was brought into the clinic suffering from shock, pale and cold, the pulse was irregular, the left side of his face was swollen and deep purple, his left eye was closed and swollen. He was given *Arnica* every 15 minutes and his face was dressed with a *Calendula* dressing. After the first dose of *Arnica* he went to sleep ; when I saw him two hours later his pulse and respiration were steady. The Sister stated that the swelling had already much improved as he had looked almost dead when he was carried into the surgery. He tried to sit up as I spoke to him and declared he felt much more himself, then he brought up some undigested food. Three hours after the accident he walked home looking greatly improved. He rested in bed for the rest of the day at his home, taking *Arnica*, 4 hourly. The swelling of the left cheek and eye was much diminished by the next morning, when he walked, jauntily, into the surgery ; the swelling of the face and eye cleared in under four days, and he was back at the milk round in time for the Saturday delivery. Surely a most satisfactory and rapid cure.

A similar case was that of a girl of about fourteen years of age who was brought in by her companions after a similar fall on the paving stones. Her features were unrecognizable, both eyes closed by the swelling. The face was a purple pulpy mass, blood streaming all over her. She was cleaned up with *Calendula*, and a cold *Calendula* dressing was applied to the face. *Arnica* was given 2 hourly at first and then 4 hourly, within two days the face had almost returned to normal. There was no sepsis and she was discharged completely cured in five days.

Arnica ointment can well be applied instead of *Arnica* lotion to bruises, contusions, etc. It is more conveniently applied than a lotion, and many people prefer it. The same precaution must be used as is mentioned under *Arnica* lotion, it should not be applied to an open wound.

Arnica thus can be used internally for bruised muscles, prevention of shock, concussion, apoplexy, falls and injuries to any part of the body. It is useful and should not be forgotten in corns due to pressure of ill-fitting footwear, given internally and applied externally.

LEDUM

The next remedy for such accidents as stabs, punctured wounds from sharp-pointed instruments as awls, rusty nails, not forgetting lancets and scalpels, bites from animals, dogs, horses, cats and rats ; insect stings, septic wounds, whitlows caused by needle pricks, splinters under nails, etc., is *Ledum*. A remedy totally unknown, to their loss, to the general run of doctors and the orthodox pharmacists, nevertheless it has proved clinically to be invaluable for such injuries. It takes the shooting and pricking pain out of these wounds, especially in those cases where the patient prefers cold dressings to hot fomentations. It prevents sepsis in the majority of these injuries, and if given early enough, it even prevents tetanus. Yes, without giving anti-tetanic serum ! *Ledum* may be given ½ hourly, hourly, 2 hourly or 4 hourly as required, according to the severity of the injury, this means *repeat whenever the pain returns*. If a horse steps on a rusty nail which goes through to the Coffin bone, the horse will die of tetanus in spite of poultices and liniments, but no tetanus will develop and the horse will live if repeated doses of *Ledum* are given. Several such cases have been reported by a doctor in North America.

A young man ran the prongs of a pitch fork into his forehead, just by the side of his nose into the soft tissues above the eye, while loading manure. Pain, shock and swelling were severe, the eye was completely closed. *Arnica* was given, though helping the shock somewhat it was not sufficient to bring complete alleviation. Some twelve hours after the accident *Ledum* was obtained and given 2 hourly and later less frequently, result : rapid aseptic healing, no tetanus, the swelling over the eye cleared in 24 hours, the pain disappeared after the first dose of *Ledum*. The young fellow returned to work in four days, disgruntled at being kept away so long, as he felt perfectly all right.

A woman some years ago ran a rusty wire into her finger under her nail. With *Ledum*, 4 hourly, and *Calendula* dressings the finger healed by first intention in two days. I treated a similar injury while I was a surgical clerk in a well-known University hospital with the usual antiseptic dressings as ordered by the chief. It went septic and took several weeks to heal in spite of the attention given by the excellent and well experienced surgeon who was in charge of the case. Such is the advantage of *Ledum* over orthodox practice.

Ledum is excellent for cases of severe bruising, black eye and extravasations of blood and hæmatomas, where *Arnica* is not sufficiently potent to absorb it. A woman patient was seen during the blitz in 1940, who had been knocked down some area steps by the explosion of a bomb, extensive bruising of the leg and minor cuts and abrasions with concussion resulted, for which she was kept in hospital for over two weeks. When I saw her after her discharge from the hospital, the injured leg was still double the size of the other from the ankle up to the knee, glistening and purple. The blood appeared as if it were ready to burst through the skin, she was unable to walk and indeed afraid to. The only advice the hospital could offer was rest, which was impossible for her, owing to her family responsibilities. *Arnica*, 3 times a day was given for three days without any effect on the size, colour or pain of the leg. *Ledum*, 3 times daily was then prescribed and three days later the pain was considerably easier, she was able to sleep and the swelling had diminished. After continuing *Ledum* for another few days the leg was normal in size and colour. Within seven days after the first dose of this remedy, she was able to walk without any trouble, indeed she had been running round for two days looking for a new home.

A striking contrast to this was a case I had dealt with some years previously when a patient slipped on the steps of the Vatican after an audience with the Pope, injuring her shin bone. When I saw her about a week later the swelling was hard, the leg was deeply pigmented half-way up. With massage, infra-red and galvanic battery twice a week the limb took eight weeks to return to normal, although the patient had ample opportunity to rest and a car to take her around everywhere. Had I known of *Ledum* in those days, how different would have been the duration of her disability. Indeed how different would it have been in my own case, where it took nearly a year for the ankle which I had sprained repeatedly and severely within a few weeks and in the end fractured, to recover and return to normal size and function. It took weeks of gentle and skilful massage, rest and months of treatment with the Bristow battery. If I had known of the dynamic power of *Ledum* in absorbing serum and blood clots there would have been no adhesions in the ankle and neighbouring tissues to disperse with the aid of the galvanic battery and massage, and I should have been saved much pain and prolonged disability.

A young girl fell from a train on to the platform, injuring the bones of her foot. The local doctor applied lead lotion externally and ordered rest while waiting for the X-ray. The parents gave *Arnica* at once and changed it later to *Ledum*, 4 hourly, on my recommendation. Much to the doctor's surprise on taking off the bandage two days later, every sign of swelling of the foot had disappeared, though the X-ray showed signs of a fractured metatarsal. *Ledum* was continued for a few days, the foot was firmly bandaged and there was no further trouble except for some slight pain on walking for a week or two.

Remember *Ledum* in punctured wounds, contusions, extravasations such as black eye, etc., injuries, where the affected part feels cold to the touch, yet is relieved by cold applications.

Hypericum

Hypericum is closely related to and follows well after *Ledum*, pain from a punctured wound begins to go up the limb, then *Hypericum* will take hold and finish the case by preventing further extension of sepsis. If a case is seen so late that early signs of lockjaw are already present—which may come on within a day or two of an injury due to particles of street dust, contaminated with horse manure, being carried into the wound—*Hypericum* will act similarly. The muscles develop cramp near the injury and later the jaw muscles become attacked, causing inability to open the mouth. Several cases have been reported where *Hypericum* given in repeated doses at 15 minutes to ½-hourly intervals cured such an alarming state in 12 hours and no antitetanic serum was required.

After-effects or injury to the coccyx, concussion of the spine and so-called railway spine respond well to *Hypericum*.

A girl was thrown on to the back of her head in the blackout; insufferable and agonizing pain at the back of the head followed. *Arnica* was given but did not help, due to the bruising of the nerves of the spinal column, for *Arnica* only acts on bruised muscles and connective tissues. *Hypericum*, being the remedy for bruised nerves, was then ordered to be taken 2 hourly; within a few minutes after the first dose, the pain eased up, and the second dose removed it entirely. " It was marvellous," she said. The local doctor at the munition factory where she was employed, who had seen her immediately after the accident and sent her home, told her it would be at least a week before she would be able to get back to work; she returned, however, fit and well in 48 hours.

Pain in the coccyx after injury at birth, sometimes due to

the bruising of the nerves round the bone, sometimes due to actual fracture of the coccyx are the despair of the gynæcologists and the psychologists, and even the removal of the coccyx by a surgeon has little effect on the local condition. These unfortunate women drag on their miserable existence for years, yet if they but knew of *Hypericum*, they could be freed from this torture—for torture it is to them—within literally a week or two. I speak from personal clinical experience. I have seen these women in Dublin, in Edinburgh, in Manchester women's hospitals, and the tale was always the same—" leave them alone, nothing can be done for them." Within the last ten years I have cured numerous sufferers with *Hypericum*, and on an average the cure took less than a fortnight.

Years ago a boy was seen with a compound fracture of the humerus. *Hypericum* was given 2 hourly for 24 hours, the arm being immobilized, then the limb was set under an anæsthetic and fixed in plaster of Paris with a window cut out to facilitate the dressing of the wound. Tincture of *Hypericum* was applied locally, *Arnica* was given 4 hourly, there was no sepsis and hardly any pain. The arm healed perfectly within three weeks.

Hypericum is also most successful for crushed fingers or toes or superficial abrasions, where sensitive nerve endings are left exposed. *Hypericum* used internally at 2 to 4 hourly intervals with *Hypericum* tincture applied locally will cure these cases rapidly. I remember a case of a livery man at some stables near the hospital who had been bitten by a fractious horse and who came up to the surgery after the usual hot fomentations had been applied for a week and failed to give any relief. His thumb was discoloured and swollen, the sepsis had spread along the palmar fascia up the arm, the axillary glands were enlarged and tender. He had a temperature of 102 degrees, tongue was coated thickly, and he was highly toxic. His hand was put in a *Hypericum* bath for half an hour, a tepid *Hypericum* dressing was applied, *Hypericum* was given ½ hourly internally, the local treatment was repeated every 4 hours ; the relief was great and rapid, temperature normal in 24 hours, the septic intoxication cleared up, and the thumb discharged freely. In a week the whole condition had disappeared, there was no stiffening of the muscles or loss of function.

One of my patients came to the dispensary with an abscess in the palmar fascia which was bulging and extremely painful. An *Hypericum* compress was applied to the hand and changed 4 hourly, it was also given internally and within 6 hours the hand was discharging freely, there was no more pain and the hand was completely healed within the week.

A young lad was brought in with a severely lacerated palm with the skin hanging down in strips. Pure *Calendula* tincture was applied to arrest the bleeding which enabled me to put in 16 stitches, making a neat patchwork of the palm. A *Hypericum* compress was applied locally and *Hypericum* given internally 4 hourly. It healed perfectly without sepsis within a week.

Hypericum is useful in all stings, punctured wounds, bites, etc., if the pain shoots up the nerves of the limb from the wound. I well remember experiencing the benefit of *Hypericum* personally when bitten on the toe by a horse fly while walking in Switzerland. A few hours later not only was the toe swollen, excessively painful and tender, but the pain and swelling had extended well beyond the ankle. I was miles away from any hospital and without any means of transport save by riding on mule back and then sitting for hours in an open coach. An infusion was made by steeping and boiling the entire plant of *Hypericum*, root included, which had been collected on the nearby mountainside. A compress was soaked in the hot infusion, wrung out and applied to the foot and renewed whenever it dried. *Hypericum* was taken internally 3 times a day and in under two days I was able to put my foot to the ground and limp about the hotel grounds. It was quite recovered in five or six days.

At least one sergeant in the 1914–18 war used *Hypericum* at the battle front for shrapnel wounds in his platoon with gratifying results. He remarked that the effect of the *Hypericum* surprised him beyond words. " To see a man badly wounded by shrapnel through his shoulder joint and in terrible pain, to be transformed to laugh and joke with the men by two little pellets is something wonderful." (Published in *The Oban Times*, May, 1915.)

Grazes and abrasions of the knee, sometimes extensive, show no signs of inflammation or sepsis after one local dressing with *Hypericum* lotion and one dose of *Hypericum* internally, 12 hours later no gravel rash follows or sepsis ; on an average the raw area is healed in 3 to 5 days, or at the worst, in a week.

Hypericum is of great use in alleviating the oft agonizing pains in an amputated limb. The stump is largely a mass of sensitive nerve-endings which, so to speak, have been left hanging in the air. *Hypericum* ointment should be applied as soon as possible after the amputation to the healing area of the stump and *Hypericum* should be given internally 4 hourly at first and then 2 or 3 times a day, or whenever the pain returns. It is a well-known fact that a patient feels pains in his fingers or toes long after the limb has been amputated. The ordinary materialistic surgeon may ascribe this sensation to wishful thinking ; the more advanced physician entrusted with a knowledge of spiritual science will give you a much more reasonable explanation, based on the invisible anatomy of the human being. This can only be hinted at here at the moment. The fact remains, however, that *Hypericum* will cure these pains better than Aspirin or even Morphia.

Therefore remember *Hypericum* for lacerations, crushed fingers and toes, injured nerves, even tetanus, also for compound fractures, falls on the coccyx however long ago, and falls on the spine anywhere.

Ruta

Just as *Arnica* acts on bruised muscles so does *Ruta*, the common garden Rue, act predominantly on torn and wrenched tendons, on split ligaments of joints and on the bruised periosteum or coverings of bones. Synovitis, inflammation of the ligaments, inflammation of the knee joints and the wrist joints will respond well to *Ruta*. Bruises and kicks on the shin in footballers and hockey players, etc., need *Ruta* for a speedy recovery and for prevention of the footballers' nodules on the shin bone. A strained tendon which usually means partial detachment of the tendon from the bone will recover more rapidly under *Ruta* than if left to nature alone. Pain after osteopathic manipulations of the spine and pelvis will disappear quickly after a dose or two of *Ruta*. A partially detached tendon can be a serious drawback to an active person as it usually means rest of some weeks' duration ; with *Ruta* and a firm elastic bandage one is able to use the limb in moderation with the minimum of discomfort and without doing harm to it as I have proved personally. Give a dose or two of *Arnica* first for the shock of the accident, followed by *Ruta* after the shock has subsided, and repeat the latter whenever the pain recurs in the torn tendon or the bruised periosteum.

Housemaid's knee, tennis elbow, ganglion of the wrist respond well to *Ruta* in potency. The swelling and limitation of movement (loss of function) and prolonged period of pain which are the effects following a Colles' or Potts' fracture will be materially improved and recovery hastened by *Ruta* every 2 to 4 hours.

Ruta ointment is of use in painful bunion and broken chilblains. To make this : leave the flowering tops of fresh Rue in hot liquid lard for some hours in a warm place until all the goodness is extracted.

Symphytum or Comfrey

Symphytum or Comfrey is another remedy which acts both on the periosteum and the bones themselves. If *Ruta* should fail to relieve periosteal pain within 24 hours, go to *Symphytum* which has a deeper action. *Symphytum* tincture applied locally as a dressing or *Symphytum* ointment will fortify the action of the *Symphytum* given internally. *Symphytum* contains a principle called allantoin which has been found to be an excellent vulnerary and was used in the 1914–18 war as it was proved to have a powerful action in promoting cell proliferation ; it was used therefore as a dressing for ulcers, chronic wounds, slow healing burns, etc., with great success. Thus confirming the statement made by our old friend Gerard, the well-known herbalist, who states that a salve concocted from the fresh herb, will certainly tend to promote the healing of the bruised and broken parts. For centuries surgeons have used dressings of Comfrey mucilage from the powdered root dissolved in water for fractured bones, because it hastens the formation of callus, so necessary for the repair of bones. The knowledge of the action of this agent was originally based on folk lore ; within the last hundred and fifty years it has been found that given internally, the healing action is even speedier.

Just a few preliminary words on the first aid diagnosis of a fracture. The list of these signs and symptoms is well known and due emphasis is laid on it, viz. : (1) pain ; (2) loss of power ; (3) swelling ; (4) deformity ; (5) unnatural mobility ; (6) tenderness and (7) shortening of limb. But the importance of shock is usually overlooked, and if the patient complains of unduly severe pain in a limb and there are signs of shock, look out for a fracture and hunt for seat of the injury. One of the elementary rules of examination is often forgotten. It should become second nature to a doctor as well as to the first-aid personnel to inspect each limb before touching it and before palpation, and always to compare it with its fellow on the opposite side, line by line. If a spot of undue tenderness is found along the course of a bone, suspect a fracture and treat it as such, until confirmed or otherwise by an X-ray—as it is laid down in the First Aid Manuals, except that in addition the medicinal treatment by means of the suitable homœopathic remedies should not be forgotten. They are most valuable in combating shock and pain.

The treatment for a fracture is as follows :

A simple fracture. Give *Arnica* immediately and repeat as required 1 to 2 to 4 hourly until the effects of shock have passed off, usually within 24 hours ; then *Ledum* 4 hourly or 3 times a day to assist the absorption of the extravasation of blood which may take three to four days, followed by *Symphytum* 3 times a day until the bone has united. The whole process under this treatment usually takes about half the time necessary for the healing of the bones under the ordinary treatment, with added comfort to the patient over the whole period. There will be no rise of temperature, no acceleration of the pulse as is usual after fractures ; the patient will sleep under the *Arnica* as well as and better than under the action of Aspirin or stronger sleeping draughts which palliate only without healing at the same time. The remedies that I have mentioned not only help to comfort the patient but expedite the healing of the injury as well and there is no fear of producing a drug craving.

For compound fractures, accompanied by the bruising of the nerves give *Hypericum* immediately to alleviate the nerve pain, repeating whenever there is return of the pain, and then, when the nerve pain has ceased, give *Arnica* for 1 to 2 days for the shock, then *Ledum*, for a few days, if there is much bruising and swelling of the softer parts covering the bone, until this has become absorbed and then finish off with *Symphytum* 3 times daily to promote the healing of the bone.

These treatments for simple and compound fractures are in addition to and not in place of the usual surgical procedures, such as setting the bone in correct alignment as confirmed by X-ray examination, proper fixation of the joints above and below the seat of fracture by means of suitable splints, immediate gentle massage by trained masseuses combined with passive movements of fingers or toes in the case of arm, wrist or leg fractures respectively, followed later by active movements of the muscles by the patient himself. This obviates the long period of rigidity of the muscles, due to adhesions as a result of their prolonged inactivity. Herein I follow the teaching of Sir Robert Jones, the first of British surgeons to advocate the study of orthopædics, and who preached the earliest possible use of the muscles even while the bones were still kept at rest.

Symphytum is also useful in injury to the eyeball and the surrounding bone (orbital periosteum) due to injury by stone or heavy stick, and will prevent cataract and ensuing blindness, as I have proved in several cases. Another injury where it proves its value is the bruising of the cheek, the periosteum of the malar bone which is as near the surface as the shin bone. A fall on the face causing extensive bruising and extravasation and discoloration of the face, produces a depressing effect on the patient, which if untreated, may persist for several weeks.

I remember two cases, both with this injury : one was treated with *Arnica* alone, the bruising and discoloration did not disappear for nearly three weeks ; the second was given *Arnica* for 24 hours and then *Symphytum*, here the pigmentation cleared up under a week.

Remember *Symphytum* for bruised periosteum and fractured bones.

RHUS TOX.

Rhus tox. is the remedy par excellence for ruptured ligaments and tendons round joints. Sprained wrists and sprained ankles are among the most common accidents, which should be treated as always with *Arnica* in repeated doses for the primary shock for about 24 to 48 hours, followed by *Ledum* for the extravasation of blood (bruising) which usually follows, and later with *Rhus tox.* 2 hourly, then 4 hourly for several days or until the patient has recovered from the sprain.   An excellent mechanical adjuvant I find is soap and water massage of the injured joint, carried out as soon after the accident as possible.   This requires a bowl of hot water, as hot as can be borne by the patient, and an ample supply of good soap.   Personally I prefer Wright's Coal Tar Soap, as it gives a very good lather.   The operator sits in front of the patient, a little to the side, placing a mackintosh and towel on her lap.   The injured limb is immersed for a few minutes in the hot water and then placed comfortably on the operator's knee, who will proceed to lather her hands thickly with the soap and with a rotary movement gently smoothe the skin round the injured joint, always keeping her hands thickly covered with lather, thus preventing any undue friction or excessive pressure of any kind.   The limb should be massaged over the injured area on both sides of the joint and the movements should extend well above and below the seat of injury.   This should be carried out for at least half an hour, not sparing the soap or allowing the water to cool.   It must also be emphasized that the limb must be supported from below throughout its entire length. This operation should be repeated once in every 24 hours and will have the effect of reducing the swelling rapidly and decreasing the pain.   I have known cases of sprained ankles of medium severity where daily soap and water massage was begun within an hour or two of the accident, and *Arnica* followed by *Rhus tox.*, as advised previously, was given, recover within three or four days so far as to be fit for a ten or twelve mile tramp in less than ten days, and without the subsequent development of rheumatic pains and a barometer joint, *i.e.*, the unfortunate joint which reacts to changes in the weather.   This rapid recovery is not the prerogative of youth as might be imagined by some questioning minds, for I recall a case many years ago of a lady well over sixty years old who was knocked down by a car and suffered a sprained ankle, contusion of the foot and fracture of one or two of the metatarsal bones and mild concussion.   She insisted on leaving the hospital as soon as she regained consciousness and going home, where I saw her immediately on her return. I gave her repeated doses of *Arnica* for the shock, daily soap and water massage for a week, followed by *Rhus tox.* 3 times a day, keeping her in bed for a period of ten days, and her room for another three or four days. Her first trip was to the radiologist for an X-ray examination of her foot. He told her that she would have a barometer foot for the rest of her life, even though the joint and the metatarsal bones had completely recovered. Time proved this prophecy false, for this reaction to the changes in the weather never developed and I was in close touch with this lady for many years, so I know this to be true.

Talking about being sensitive to the changes in the weather reminds me of the vital action that *Rhus tox.* has in curing certain types of rheumatism of the muscles including lumbago, which is rheumatism of the back muscles ; also fibrositis, rheumatic joints, etc., where the outstanding symptoms are stiffness and pain on beginning to move, ameliorated by continued motion and affected by changes in the weather. The cause of these being traceable to a preliminary soaking or living in a damp house or near a water course where there is frequent rising of mists.

In old sprains neglected in so far that they have not had the treatment here described, you will find a certain weakness of the affected joints. In these cases a few doses of *Calc. carb.* will rectify the remaining stiffness and weakness, especially if the sufferers are heavy individuals inclined to overweight, with puffy, clammy feet, who as a rule are easily affected by cold or changes in temperature.

Calc. phos. will help in those cases where there is easy dislocation and constant turning over of the ankles or spraining of the wrist. It should be given 3 times a day for a week or two, which usually arrests the weakness of the affected joints.

Remember, therefore, *Rhus tox.* for sprains and strains of muscles.

DISLOCATIONS

A Dislocation of a joint should be reduced as soon as possible after the accident has occurred and X-rayed to verify the correct readjustment of the joint. Of course for immediate shock and pain *Arnica* should be given internally and repeated whenever the pain is troublesome, 3 to 4 hourly and less often after a day or two. This should be carried on for 8 to 10 days at least. The patient will have good nights under the action of the *Arnica*. I have more than once deceived a patient into believing they were having Morphia, when all they had was a dose of *Arnica* before going to sleep. One lady used to be pleasantly surprised that she did not wake up with such a thick head as she did when she had Morphia on previous occasions. No further medicinal treatment is required. Massage and passive active movements should be carried out as ordered by the surgeon. *Rhus tox.* should be given 4 hourly for dislocations of the lower jaw.

TREATMENT OF WOUNDS

THE first-aider and the man in the street look upon Iodine as the preventive and cure-all for any and all varieties of sepsis, as he has been taught to do for several decades. He usually interprets the instruction of applying Iodine for any breach of the skin by thickly painting it for inches round the cut or abrasion, however minute it may be. I have seen a whole arm covered with Iodine for a skin lesion barely half an inch in length. Iodine burns and tans the epithelial cells and devitalizes them, thus allowing any septic organisms which may be lurking in the skin to attack this almost dead patch of iodized integument. Many people are extremely sensitive to the action of Iodine and constitutional symptoms may follow its application ; and other antiseptics, such as the various Lysol substitutes which are almost household words now, are not much better. In my opinion, and from my experience, it is much safer to leave the Iodine brush and bottle and antiseptics as a whole, including surgical spirit, severely alone and depend entirely on aseptic methods. Wash the broken skin under a tap of running water if available, this will wash away particles of dirt and septic organisms ; if no running water is available, always wash AWAY from the wound with clean rags dipped in cold boiled water and soap, and never, never swab inwards towards the wound. If the skin is very oily, greasy and dirty, such as is likely to be the case in a man or woman who works in a machine shop, use cotton wool and turpentine to clean off the worst of the grease, remembering to wipe the dirt off in a direction away from the wound. When the tissues surrounding the wound are reasonably clean apply *Calendula* lotion as a dressing, either in the form of a diluted tincture or the *Succus Calendulae*, the fresh plant juice. The disadvantage of the latter is that it does not keep very long once the bottle has been opened. Both these can be obtained from any good homœopathic chemist. *Calendula* is the most satisfactory wound dressing I have come across and I have tried a good many.

Scientific medicine bases its theories and treatments on mass control observations and statistics based on them. For fifteen years, as Medical Officer at a Surgical Out-Patients Centre, I have seen and watched the effects of various antiseptic dressings on many varieties of wounds, ulcers, sores, etc., seeing on an average more than 80 cases a week, and I have never been satisfied that I got hold of the ideal antiseptics. For the last five years I have broken away from my conservative habits and have used instead various plant tinctures and ointments impregnated with them. The numbers attending the centre fell owing to war conditions, evacuation, etc., but I still saw about 40 cases a week and averaged 2,000 cases a year. On these figures I consider I am entitled to base my conclusions that the methods I now employ are superior to the older and more generally accepted ones ; for these cases have yielded much better results, 95 per cent. of them are cured and fit for discharge under a fortnight, while in the old days it was the exception to discharge any case within the specified two weeks. I mention this period, for after this time the parents were asked to pay a nominal fee.

Calendula officinalis is not an antiseptic in the true meaning of the word, but germs do not thrive in its presence. It inhibits their growth I find, and even when wounds are already badly infected I have seen offensive purulent discharges become clean and sweet smelling in a day or two, and in the rare cases where it does not answer so quickly there are other plant tinctures to take its place, of which I will speak later. *Calendula* is wonderfully soothing as an external application. It neither destroys nor irritates any new epithelial cells which are growing ; on the contrary it stimulates their growth. The *Calendula* tincture is diluted for use by adding one teaspoonful to a pint of boiled water, but lately I have found that ordinary unboiled water will do just as well. Oh ! shades of my venerable teachers of Surgery, in my " Alma Mater," may I be forgiven for this heresy ; but I stick to it in spite of my strict upbringing in antisepsis and asepsis ! *Calendula* inhibits the growth of micro-organisms, why therefore bother to boil the water ; yet it is so, pus will never make its appearance in a clean wound and will disappear rapidly in an infected wound if *Calendula* is used as a dressing. If the wound is deep, one can syringe with *Calendula* and pack it lightly with gauze soaked in *Calendula*, covering the wound with dry gauze, cotton wool and bandage. The wounds in the majority of cases need only to be dressed once a day, unless they are very acute and there is much inflammation present. In some cases in order to prevent the gauze sticking to ulcers and raw areas it is left on and moistened with the lotion whenever it becomes dry ; by this method the wounds and ulcers heal more rapidly than with any other antiseptics I have tried. My pen has run away with me—this really applies for dressings of war wounds, ulcers, septic fingers, etc., and not merely to first-aid dressings. It may, however, be of interest and help to those who have to deal with local conditions and septic wounds of all kinds.

Calendula dressings were used in the American Civil War by a number of surgeons who warmly recommended their use. A Mr. Carleton, a surgeon of one of the large hospitals in the United States of America, used *Calendula* for all his operation cases, both for abdominal and bone surgery and published his results in a book, giving ample evidence of the efficacy of *Calendula* in surgery. Yet another American doctor in the 1914–18 war worked as head surgeon in one of the field hospitals under the jurisdiction of the French Army. I refer to Dr. Petrie Hoyle. Indeed he received high praise from a visiting staff officer for the clean state of the patients' wounds, the absence of smell in the wards and was congratulated on the rapid evacuation of cured cases from the hospital and the low mortality rate. I am therefore not unique in my appreciation of *Calendula* as a first-class dressing for wounds ; my only regret is that it is not better known and more widely used.

Everybody should grow *Calendula* or common Marigold on any spare patch of garden they have ; it grows easily, the golden flowers give a patch of welcome colour these grim days, besides being a most useful plant medicinally. The half-open buds or newly opened flowers with the gummy end shoots are the parts used for the tincture or the Succus. These buds and flowers should be pounded and macerated in 50 per cent. alcohol—if you use stronger alcohol the valuable balsams in the plant will coagulate—and placed in corked bottles which should be shaken several times a day for three weeks to extract all the ingredients, then remove the clear fluid by filtration and keep this tincture as stock.

The fresh plant juice or Succus is made by pulping the buds and flowers and soaking them in warm, not hot, water for 12 hours, when the lotion is ready for use ; add a small quantity of alcohol if you want to preserve the liquid for a short period of time.

The fresh yellow florets of the flowers can be applied directly to the wound and covered with a bandage ; or the pulped fresh blooms can be applied and bound over the wound. This method answers particularly well in all kinds of insect stings, bees, wasps, etc.

Calendula ointment is extremely soothing and heals rapidly when applied to all kinds of cuts, cracks, chapped hands and legs, small septic spots, etc. It is of much greater value than the ubiquitous boracic, zinc or calamine ointments. It can easily be made at home by melting such fats as spermaceti, if obtainable, or lanolin or even mutton fat with a few drops of olive or castor oil in it, in an earthenware pot, such as a 2-lb. marmalade jar, standing it in a saucepan of boiling water. Add a drachm of *Calendula* tincture to half a pound of melted fat, stirring it with a spatula after the heat has been turned off, continuing to stir vigorously while the fat is solidifying. If successful, there will be no trace of the *Calendula* tincture at the bottom of the jar. Olive or castor oil should be added to the liquified mutton fat in the proportion of half teaspoonful of oil to half pound of fat at the same time as the *Calendula* tincture ; for the cold mutton fat is too hard to be applied to the skin directly.

A case that came to my notice recently which showed the healing property of *Calendula* ointment was that of a woman with a splinter, broken off and left under the nail for 12 hours, this was removed by cutting down the nail with a sharp scalpel under cocaine. The *Calendula* ointment was applied, and one dose of *Ledum* given, the pain disappeared at once and the finger healed without any further trouble in 12 hours. The remark the patient made was that she had had many splinters removed at various times, but never with so little pain during the removal or afterwards, which speaks for itself.

Although I have sung the praises of *Calendula*, I would not ignore or forget the almost equal virtues of *Hypericum* as a vulnerary ; indeed I interchange them sometimes if there is one or other in short supply. One of the most rapid cases of the healing of a lacerated lip and a deep cut over the bridge of the nose, which I have seen, was a lady of eighty-four, who injured herself in getting out of bed by falling against some furniture. *Hypericum* lotion was applied to the lips and to the cut on the nose, which were both healed within a few hours, leaving no scar whatsoever ; no stitches were put in, merely an *Hypericum* dressing over the cuts.

Hypericum tincture is made in a similar manner as the *Calendula* tincture, and the *Hypericum* ointment also. There is, however, an alternative method of preparation by taking a large handful of the *Hypericum* flowers and placing them in olive oil and stirring them over gentle heat for half an hour while all the " goodness " is extracted, the flowers are then removed and the oil is allowed to cool. This *Hypericum* oil is wonderfully soothing and healing for all kinds of sores. On the whole, I prefer *Hypericum* for highly septic wounds, whitlows, septic nails, cellulitis, gangrenous toes, ulcers and so on. Herein you follow on the same lines as already given in the chapter on the internal administration of *Hypericum* : that is, it is most useful in those painful conditions where the shooting pains extend from the seat of injury.

A headmaster came for treatment for a septic finger, which he had tried to cure for a fortnight with Boracic fomentations and later Magnesium sulphate applications, without any effect whatsoever ; the pain and sepsis increasing in severity rather than decreasing. When I saw the whitlow I was afraid that his finger would become permanently stiff because of the threatened sloughing of the tendon. *Hypericum* dressings were applied twice daily and he was given *Silica* internally 3 times a day—*Silica* because of the history of long sepsis without any crushing or laceration of the parts. The finger started to discharge after the first application of *Hypericum* and in three days it was healed. There was no need to open the inflamed area, there was no loss of function, and he was extremely grateful for the rapid improvement and the cessation of pain.

For external applications to boils and carbuncles I prefer

Hypericum to *Calendula* and wherever there is extensive laceration of the tissues. A young lad came to me who had cut his shin against some paving stones, the wound was gaping and he complained of great pain. It was cleaned up with 1 in 25 *Hypericum* and a *Hypericum* dressing was applied, firmly strapped across. It was healed in two days.

I remember the case of a man in hospital who had had an accident to his leg which had torn the attachments of the muscles from the Tibia (shin bone) for about six inches. The wound was cleansed with *Hypericum* while the man was under an anæsthetic, and after the tissues were replaced a *Hypericum* dressing was applied and strapped across firmly in position. This was not removed but *Hypericum* lotion was applied between the strappings. The wound was healed and the man discharged from hospital in a week able to walk with only a slight limp which disappeared in due course.

I have used *Hypericum* in so many cases that it would be just a repetition of what has been said already. Now for a practical hint. These plant tinctures are expensive to buy in the first instance due to the high cost of the alcohol used in the making and the cost of collecting and preparing them. They are, however, extremely economical in use as only a few drops are required, the same with the ointments. A teaspoonful of tincture will medicate half-pound of ointment base. The ointment should be applied with care and in moderation.

HÆMORRHAGE

THE usual first - aid instructions as regards Hæmorrhage should be used, such as local compressions and, where necessary, tourniquets above the bleeding point, with the usual precaution of loosening the tourniquets at 15 minute intervals at least to allow the blood to flow through the limb until the patient reaches the hospital where the ligaturing of the torn blood vessels can be attended to. But I can give a few hints on how to stop minor hæmorrhages rapidly by a simple first-aid method, a method which is at present almost unknown. The first time I tried it out the result was most dramatic.

A builder who was working on some demolition works near the surgery was brought along with capillary hæmorrhage from the back of the hand, due to scraping it against some stones ; his fellow workmen had applied the usual first-aid methods of local compression for more than half an hour without any result whatsoever. His bandages were soaked through the moment they were applied in spite of putting on thick pads of cotton wool and bandage. When he was finally brought to me at the surgery I reached for the bottle of *Calendula* tincture and found to my dismay that it was empty except for a few scanty drops at the bottom. I just dripped these precious droplets over the bleeding back of the hand and hoped and prayed that there would be sufficient to meet the requirements. The result was instantaneous. The bleeding stopped, as if somebody had used a charm. I watched for ten minutes, and as there was no return of the oozing a dry dressing was applied firmly over the wounded area and bandaged in position ; no further trouble ensued. The nursing staff have used pure *Calendula* tincture ever since in all cases of external hæmorrhages and it never fails to act. Let me give a further example or two.

A lad came along one day with a large triangular cut on the back of one of his fingers which was bleeding profusely. Various people had tried to stop the bleeding for an hour but without any success ; it went on spouting. He looked pale and frightened. Sister tried to encourage him by assuring him she could stop the bleeding at once, he was just to watch for the miracle. She dabbed on pure *Calendula,* just a drop or two ; the boy looked on hardly believing his eyes, when hey presto ! the bleeding ceased. The two or three schoolfellows who had brought him were craning their necks to look on, their ejaculations of " Blimey, Sister, it's stopped," bore witness to the fact, the truth of which had to be seen to be believed. She then applied a *dry* gauze dressing with a covering of lint and bandaged it firmly, and when I saw it the next day it had healed completely, there was no sign of the severe hæmorrhage, no sepsis and we had no further trouble.

The first time I was told about the efficacy of *Calendula* tincture in arresting hæmorrhage was when I attended the first confinement of a young married woman, who was by pro-fession a veterinary nurse. She told me that before she could settle down to the serious business of having her own baby she must see to the docking of the tails of four pedigree pups that she had delivered four days previously and which could not be left any longer. So I held up the blind shivering bits of puppy-hood, one by one, while she snipped off the tails and applied pure *Calendula* to the bleeding areas which ceased to bleed as soon as the *Calendula* touched the surface. After this important business was over the lady retired to bed and we proceeded with the next act of presenting her husband with a lusty son and heir.

Mr. Carleton in his work on Medical and Surgical methods describes the rapid action of *Calendula* in arresting hæmorrhage from the gums. The dentist in working on Mr. Carleton's teeth had cut the gums accidentally a number of times and refused to go on with the work as the gum was so swollen ; he wanted to put on some iodine and finish the work the next day. Mr. Carleton sent out for some tincture of *Calendula,* to which he added an equal quantity of very hot water and started to rinse out his mouth. In ten minutes the gums were so reduced in size that the dentist could finish the job he had in hand ; hot water alone would not have stopped the bleeding and reduced the swelling under half an hour. Mr. Carleton adds as a corollary that it was due to the *Calendula* that the hæmorrhage and swelling ceased in ten minutes and that he had further proofs of its power in many other instances.

Now for a few more incidents which happened in my work at the surgical centre.

A boy was almost carried in by his school friends, collapsed and faint as the result of being knocked out by the water waste-preventer falling on his head, while pulling the plug in the school lavatories. It had become unsafe from the vibration of the bombing. His scalp was deeply cut for some inches ; there were quantities of blood everywhere which the Sister traced to its source and then applied some *Calendula* tincture with a wooden applicator padded with cotton wool. As usual the bleeding stopped at once. She covered the cut with a *dry* gauze dressing first and then cut the hair round and cleaned off the traces of blood from the rest of the scalp ; she then strapped the dressing in position. No washing of the wound was attempted or anti-septic cleansing, only the blood was removed from the scalp after the application of the Calendula to the cut. *Arnica* was given 2 hourly, and the boy was seen 2 hours later in order to have the wound inspected. It healed without any trouble, without any sepsis or return of the hæmorrhage ; indeed when I saw it the next day there was hardly any scar visible and the boy showed no ill effects from his accident of the previous day.

A young hoyden of a girl, minute in stature but mighty in valour, had her head cut open by one of her schoolmates heaving a brick at her. The cut was two inches long and of course bleeding profusely. Young Mary came, accompanied by a gang of twelve girl friends, screaming lustily at the top of her voice Again Sister did not do any washing or thorough cleansing of the scalp. She found the seat of the injury, applied the pure *Calendula* on cotton wool wrapped round a thin stick ; the bleeding stopped, to the great excitement of the admiring crowd of school-girl friends ; the blood was then washed off the head, a neat strand of hair was cut out in order to make room for the strapping and Mary walked off smiling, happily sucking a pill of *Arnica*, the heroine of the party. She returned in two hours' time for an inspection. Result : a perfect healing in record time.

Another case. A boy came in with a triangular cut in the

palm of his hand at the base of the third and fourth fingers, a deep gaping wound bleeding profusely. Pure *Calendula* was applied as usual without any previous washing or cleansing of the raw, exposed area of the palm, the skin flap was pulled over and a *dry* gauze dressing was applied, a layer of white lint was strapped on over it and a bandage was put on top. *Arnica* was given and he was inspected 2 hours later. No sepsis followed and the hæmorrhage did not recur. In this case the healing was somewhat slow owing to the free mobility of the hand and the habits of the neighbourhood, which consist in removing bandages and inspecting injuries ; the parents being the worst offenders.

Now, a last case, in order to emphasize the importance of putting on a dry dressing after the application of the *Calendula* to arrest bleeding. A boy came for treatment, having sliced off the top of his finger plus a piece of nail. Pure *Calendula* was applied and a *wet* dressing put on inadvertently ; the boy came back twice within three hours with a blood-soaked dressing. The Sister in charge was puzzled why the *Calendula* should have failed to arrest the bleeding. At his third visit she changed the wet dressing to the customary dry one which proved to be effective at the fourth and last visit two hours later. No sepsis followed, the finger healed perfectly in a day or two.

DENTAL HÆMORRHAGE

Hæmorrhage from the dental sockets after teeth extraction can be most alarming. Our usual procedure after extraction was to give each child a dose of *Phosphorus* when leaving the dental chair, which was repeated every 10 to 15 minutes, until there was a cessation of the bleeding, usually one or two doses were sufficient to achieve this result. In five years more than 11,000 cases were treated in this manner and we did not have any cases of hæmorrhage coming back the following day for treatment of persistent hæmorrhage ; while in the previous years when no *Phosphorus* was given it was no uncommon thing for Sister to have to stay behind for several hours to deal with one or two hæmorrhage cases out of a number of thirty or more per session. The custom in those days was to use the usual styptics and in severe cases resort to plugging the cavities. The dental surgeon and the

sister were most satisfied with the action of the *Phosphorus* as a
medicinal styptic (arrest of hæmorrhage). It saved a great deal
of anxiety and lessened their labours considerably, it also saved
them from the wrath of parents who felt that the dentist was
personally to blame if bleeding occurred. I did not know of the
styptic action of *Calendula* then, or I should have used it in addition
to the internal dosing with the *Phosphorus*, I know now that we
should have had even fewer cases of prolonged hæmorrhage
after extractions and that not more than one dose of *Phosphorus*
would have been necessary.

Nose Bleeding

The usual method of first aid of applying cold over the nose
and the spine at the level of the collar, preferably a cold key,
and putting the feet in hot water may act reasonably well, but
I find that a diluted preparation of *Vipera*, specially prepared
from the poison sac of the English common viper, is much more
efficacious. Repeat *Vipera* every quarter of an hour until the
bleeding has ceased. This is a remedy which should be used in
the 12th potency.

For Passive Bleeding from Varicose Veins

With the leg up at right angles to the body and the patient
lying down, applying a bandage on both sides of the bleeding
vein. In addition give *Hamamelis* every quarter of an hour at first,
later lengthening the intervals until the bleeding has stopped.
Two or three doses at the most should be sufficient to achieve
this. If the patient is a thin, shrivelled up elderly woman and
the blood is dark, almost black and watery, *Secale* given every
quarter or half hour, until the bleeding ceases, will answer better.

For Internal Hæmorrhage

If from the lungs or stomach, the patient requires to be under
expert medical advice and should be admitted to a hospital, but
until he is admitted it may be possible to try the effects of such
a remedy as *Ferrum phos.* in repeated doses, or *Ipecacuanha* if the

hæmorrhage is bright and gushing, or *Aconite* if the patient is extremely restless and shows evidence of extreme fright and fear of death. *Arnica* may help, if *Ipecacuanha* fails.

For the after effects of hæmorrhage, when the patient is pale, white and bloodless, feels cold and shivery, is extremely weak and easily exhausted, *China* in 4 hourly doses will quickly put such a person on to the road to health and restore the iron to the red blood corpuscles. In a few cases, where the loss has been extreme and the patient is much debilitated and there is little hæmatin in the blood, material doses of iron may be necessary, the best preparation of iron in my opinion is *Ferrum protoxalate*, 2 grains of the 1x potency, 3 times daily, extended over several weeks. The hæmoglobin content of the blood will rise steeply within a short time after its administration. I know the fashion is to use the Blood Bank and replace the blood lost through hæmorrhage, or in any weakened debilitated condition by transfusion of blood. There are various serious factors to be considered in this procedure. Blood, as the vehicle of life, is specific to each individual, containing properties peculiar to each person ; aggravations and conflicts, physical, mental and spiritual, are likely to ensue when foreign blood is introduced. We know not what the ultimate outcome will be, a total change of personality is likely. Subcutaneous salines and intravenous salines, plus *China* and Iron salts have saved many lives in the past in an acute emergency. I understand transfusion of blood is practised in cases of severe shock, where *Arnica* would do as well if not better, if this action of *Arnica* were only sufficiently known and tried out. This is too long and serious a subject to be dealt with in a few short phrases, but I feel the words of Christ may well be applied here : " What does it profit a man if he gain the whole world and lose his own soul," or as the philosopher and poet Goethe says in Faust : " If I possess his blood, I possess the man, . . ."

FAINTING—SYNCOPE

FAINTING is due to the sudden failing of the action of the heart. It may be due to hæmorrhage, to fatigue, want of food, badly ventilated or crowded rooms, to sudden emotion, fear, bad news, sudden relief from anxiety or fear after a period of tension ; tight collar or tight clothing may be an exciting factor. Treatment : put the patient down flat, keep the head low, loosen the clothes, especially round the neck and waist, keep plenty of air space round the patient, prevent people from crowding round. If a man or young boy faints at the sight of blood make him sit down and put his head gently between his knees. These simple rules will usually help to restore a fainting person. Fainting due to long standing, processions and crowds associated with a long period of fasting, is quickly remedied by hot drinks, hot soup, tea or coffee, as soon as the patient recovers consciousness. Sudden fear associated with restlessness, feeling of fright and anxiety is put right by *Aconite*. Fainting from sudden joy, such as the return of the prodigal, is soon relieved by *Coffea*. Fainting from grief and from sudden bad news, requires *Ignatia*. Fainting from apprehensiveness and fear and fright with twitching of limbs and hysterical fits, with red face and perspiration will require *Opium* in small doses. Effects of fear and fright producing trembling of the limbs with frequency of micturition and diarrhœa needs *Gelsemium*.

EPILEPSY

No treatment should be attempted during an attack except for loosening tight garments and putting the handle of a toothbrush or pencil between the back teeth to prevent the tongue being bitten. See to it if you can that the patient does not injure himself by falling in the fire, etc., or choking, by turning him on his back. Such a patient requires prolonged medical treatment.

SUNSTROKE

For prevention in hot climates or unaccustomed exposure to the sun, attend to the state of the bowels, avoid alcohol entirely, at any rate before " sundown," and all excess in smoking and food. Excessive exercise should not be taken in the heat of the day when the sun is at its zenith. The back of the head and the top of the spine should be well protected, a large hat and a lined pith helmet should be worn in the tropics and a spinal pad lined with red cloth to intercept the actinic rays of the sun.

The symptoms are severe headache, hot dry skin, drowsiness and frequent micturition. Treatment : the patient should be kept quiet in a darkened shady place, the clothes should be loosened, a cloth should be wrung out in hot water and wrapped around the head, changing the cloth frequently, the whole body should be sponged with warm water. The best medicinal remedy is *Glonoine*, for the intense congestion of the head, the giddiness and the rush of blood to the head and chest, violent throbbing pain in the head relieved from uncovering it. *Glonoine* once or twice daily or to be repeated when throbbing returns.

Belladonna is another remedy for throbbing headache, which is made worse by lying down, giddiness when stooping, throbbing aggravated from uncovering the head or having the hair cut. *Gelsemium* for less acute fever with little delirium and the headache at the nape of the neck, face is dusky, flushed and he looks stupid and besotted, with a hot dry skin.

BURNS AND SCALDS

A GREAT deal can be achieved by the proper first-aid treatment for burns and scalds. One of the requirements is the careful removal of any clothing from a burned or scalded area; large or smaller pieces of skin may have been torn off in an effort to ease the agonies of the burned person. If the clothing should adhere to the burn, cut round it carefully, leaving the portion of clothing over the burnt area in position, to be removed by a doctor or experienced person later.

If the burn is on an exposed part of the body apply immediately a large piece of fluffy and warmed cotton wool, taking care that you do not burn the cotton wool in the process of warming it and seeing that the piece is sufficiently large to cover the entire burned area. Bandage it so that all air is excluded. The ordinary, minor domestic burns will not blister if treated in this manner, but be careful to leave the cotton wool and bandage on for several hours. If pain is troublesome, give *Urtica urens* internally, repeating it whenever the pain returns.

If a blister has already formed be careful not to break it, applying *Urtica urens* locally. A teaspoonful of the tincture is added to a pint of water or twenty drops to a large cup of water. Soak a pad of gauze in this lotion, which must be large enough to cover the area, apply to the burn, cover with lint, cotton wool and bandage. Remove the lint whenever the dressing feels dry and resoak the gauze by moistening it with a few drops of the *Urtica urens* lotion. In severe burns the *Urtica urens* may have to be applied every two or three hours. *Urtica urens* should be given internally whenever there is a return of the pain, as I have said before. *Urtica urens* relieves the pain, I have found, in approximately 7 minutes and its action may last anything from 2 to 4 and as long as 12 hours. Whenever a sudden pang of pain reminds you of the burn repeat the *Urtica urens* internally. I heard a doctor recommend the application of raw white of egg by painting it over the burn with a brush, renewing the application in 12 hours ; he claims to have achieved marvellous results in stopping the pain and healing the burns and preventing sepsis. I do not know how many people would be willing to sacrifice eggs for this treatment, either for themselves or anybody else. It might be worth while trying it. Personally *Urtica urens* internally and externally and the other measures I shall recount, have served me sufficiently well that I prefer to keep my egg as a treat for breakfast.

In more severe cases of burning where there is great pain and restlessness, blister formation or a burn of the second or even third degree, I have used *Causticum* internally and *Hypericum* lotion externally, as before soaking the gauze dressing whenever it became dry, thus preventing any tearing off of the newly formed epithelial cells and allowing undisturbed growth to take place under cover of the dressing. The *Causticum* removes the agonies of the pain within 7 to 10 minutes and should be repeated whenever the pain returns, it might be ½ hourly or 2 hourly ; the intervals between the doses lengthening as the pain improved. Now for some illustrations.

In my first year of general practice I was called out in a hurry to a case near by of a little boy under two, who had pulled a cup of scalding tea over his right arm. I heard his screams of pain as I rushed up the stairs to the room, his sleeves had been torn off and part of his skin with it. He would not let me touch it. The first thing I did was to give him a dose of *Causticum* ; in 7 minutes, as I timed it, the shrieks ceased and he allowed me to apply a dressing of *Hypericum* to the scalded area. Having made him comfortable, to the great relief of his parents, I left instructions with them to repeat the medicine whenever he started to moan or cry out, and when I called the next morning he had had a comparatively comfortable night, only needing his medicine every 4 hours. The gauze dressing was left on for a week, just moistened with the *Hypericum* when it became dry, about four or five times during the day. *Causticum* was continued 4 hourly. The burn extended from his shoulder to below his elbow, two-thirds round the arm ; it healed without sepsis in ten days without any contraction of the skin, only with the usual slight pigmentation of the skin. He never owed me a grudge for treating him, for he had never been hurt.

While I was still medical officer at the hospital I compared the results of treating burns with Picric acid and *Urtica urens* on cases of similar severity. One man came to out-patients with scalding of both his legs. The more superficial burn I treated with Picric acid and the deeper one with *Urtica urens* ; I found that the *Urtica urens* burn was three days in advance of the one treated with Picric acid, even though it was the deeper one, and the patient declared that the *Urtica urens* side was much more comfortable than the other. After trying these methods out in half a dozen cases, I came to the conclusion that I achieved better results with *Urtica urens* than with Picric acid. Henceforth I gave up the use of Picric acid entirely.

Another case of burning stays in my mind. A four-year-old boy was sitting in the hearth before an open fire in his dressing gown prior to going to bed while his aunt went outside to warm him some milk, the next moment she heard a shriek and on rushing into the room she found the child in the fire. On tearing off the pyjama legs they found the thigh burnt along its entire length, some of the skin was, of course, torn off as well. Father applied the Tannic acid jelly at once and came for me. The child was screaming with pain and fright. *Causticum* was given immediately ; again in 7 minutes the pain subsided so that I was able to have a look at the burned leg. I left the Tannic acid jelly on this burn and on further examination I found another burned patch on the abdomen, three inches by two inches, which fortunately had not been discovered. *Urtica urens* lotion was applied to this patch which was to be remoistened the moment it became dry, and *Causticum* was to be given in the night whenever he started to whimper and complain of pain. Six doses were necessary, given at 2 hourly intervals. Later the intervals were lengthened between the doses as the pain subsided. The abdominal burn which was treated with *Urtica urens* from the start healed up without any trouble, no sepsis occurred ; the burn on the thigh treated with Tannic acid jelly turned septic, although I replaced the Tannic acid on the second day with *Hypericum* lotion. It was very slow in healing ; of course the boy was spoilt and the dressings were not always applied correctly as he made so much fuss and bother. We had to change the dressing to Saline for a few days, then we applied

Calendula ointment outside the edges of the burn and *Calendula* lotion over the septic area. In four weeks the burn was healed. I consider that Tannic acid was to blame for causing the sepsis and retarding the healing.

An extensive burn (second degree) was seen four days after the right foot had been scalded with boiling water. The area extended along the outer side of the foot from heel to the third toe and over the instep and was already very septic, the dead skin lying in a crumpled heap in the middle, the whole foot being wrapped up in a dirty sock. The dead skin was removed with forceps, and without cleaning the septic burn, gauze soaked in *Hypericum* was applied over the whole area and *Calendula* ointment round the edges. *Urtica urens* was given internally. The patient came three times the first day, which greatly improved the septic condition. He was a most irregular attender, only coming when it pleased him. In spite of this he got on very well, and when I saw the burned foot some ten days later it was well on the way to recovery. The *Urtica urens* internally and the *Hypericum* was continued for three weeks.

A girl came with a second degree burn of the right wrist about four inches by three. *Urtica urens* was given and *Hypericum* applied as sepsis had already started, *Calendula* ointment being applied to the edges of the burn. The wrist was healed without any further trouble in a fortnight.

The Sister at the clinic some years ago had an accident with a large bottle of Lysol which exploded and ran over her face. The left side of her face was badly burnt and she suffered from severe shock. When she was taken home, *Hypericum* lotion was applied on gauze pads which were continually moistened, covering the whole of the left side of the face including the eyes. *Causticum* was given 2 hourly. By the next morning she had completely recovered ; there was no sign of a burn on her face, save a minute area of redness near the outer angle of the left eye, and she returned to her work none the worse for her alarming experience. This rapid recovery after a Lysol burn on such a sensitive and vital part as the face, stands out in sharp relief from the experience I had with a doctor colleague of mine years ago, who burned her forearm with Lysol. She was shocked and dazed after the accident, the arm was red, inflamed and blistered, and though she had the best treatment that could be provided at the hospital at which she was resident surgical officer, it was nearly a fortnight before she was back at her job.

For burns of the third degree—that is the severest type of burns—I find the most useful remedy is *Cantharides*, which should be given really in all cases of extensive burns, burns of the abdomen, the chest and the face, whenever there is extreme shock. These cases are liable to be followed by secondary pneumonia or duodenal ulceration due to the absorption of toxins from the injury, and the disturbance of the nitrogen balance. Dysuria (painful micturition) is often present in these cases due to the increased urinary output of nitrogen. Spraying of the extensively burned areas with a few drops of *Cantharides* 1*x* in water are well worth a trial, especially if combined with *Cantharides* internally.

Radiation with the infra-red lamp I have found a great help in the later healing stages of extensive burns ; it stimulates the growth of the epithelial cells and prevents and absorbs disfiguring scars. At least that was my experience in the cases where I was able to apply it. *Calendula* ointment applied round the edges of the burns and over the healing burns in the last stages of recovery, expedites the healing process.

Summary. For burns of first and not too extensive second degree, use *Urtica urens* internally and externally. For second degree burns : *Hypericum* externally and *Causticum* internally, and in the later stages *Calendula* lotion and *Calendula* ointment as the skin begins to grow over the raw area. For third degree burns, *Cantharides* internally in frequent doses at first, while the pain and shock are severe and less frequently when the pain is easing, also *Cantharides* externally. Later when healing has started apply *Hypericum* or *Calendula*, alternating them every few days, as soon as there seems to be a standstill in the healing process.

FOREIGN BODIES IN THE EYES

FOR foreign bodies in the eyes first see to it that the patient does not rub the eye; pull down the lower eyelid and remove the speck, if seen, with a piece of cotton wool or with the slightly wetted corner of a clean handkerchief. A foreign body under the upper eyelid requires more expert handling as the lid has to be everted. Stand behind the patient, pressing the head against your chest, place a match or surgical probe on the upper eyelid half an inch above the edge and press back as far as possible, then pull the eyelashes over it in an upward direction. This will expose the under surface of the upper eyelid, and allows for the removal of the foreign body with cotton wool. Then apply, after removal of foreign body, a weak 1 in 25 *Calendula* tincture, washing the eye in an eyebath or an undine. After this put on *Calendula* ointment on cotton wool, wrapped round the unused end of a match or surgical probe, smearing the ointment gently along the eyelids from the nasal end to the outer edge, and give *Aconite* internally.

For quicklime in the eye, the eye needs to be bathed in vinegar and water, 1 in 4, to antidote the action of the alkali. Then use *Calendula* ointment and give *Aconite* for shock.

For accidental injury to the eye with corrosive acid, bathe it with a solution of baking soda, a dessertspoonful to a pint of cold water; after which apply *Calendula* ointment and *Aconite* internally. If a foreign body should be embedded in the eyeball, before removing it pull down the lower eyelid, drop in Castor oil on the eyeball, tell the patient to close the lids, cover the eye with a large pad of cotton wool and bandage it firmly. Give *Aconite* internally.

FOREIGN BODIES IN THE EARS

SOME children are fond of placing such things as beads, stones, shells and peas into the openings of the body, particularly the ears and nose. A foreign body in the nose usually requires the aid of a doctor, unless you can make the child sneeze by making it sniff up some soap powder or snuff mixture. The effort of sneezing may expel the foreign body, unless it is pushed up too high. If there is any bleeding after the sneezing, apply a little *Calendula* ointment up the nostril.

A foreign body in the ear, if this is an insect, earwig, etc., may be removed by filling the ear with oil, preferably olive oil, which will make the insect float up to the surface handy for removal ; other foreign bodies should not be interfered with by a lay person as it may lead to serious consequences. A doctor or nurse will be able to syringe the ear with the necessary powerful metal syringe. A glass syringe should not be used. Peas or beans must not be syringed, as they will swell up and become fixed. These extraneous bodies should be removed by a doctor.

I have come across several cases where deafness in one ear was due to a shell or bead being placed in the ear canal in childhood, forgotten and left there for thirty years or longer, only to be found after syringing, embedded in the wax which had formed over it.

EARACHE

Earache may be an emergency which requires prompt treatment. It comes on after a sore throat, inflammation of the throat due to the inflammation travelling up the Eustachian tube or it may be due to reflex pain from the teeth, especially in teething children or young adults when the large molars, specially the wisdom teeth, are coming through. In earache due to an erupting tooth, put in a drop or two of tincture of *Plantago* into the ear. This is heated by putting a teaspoon into hot water

45

and dropping the *Plantago* into the spoon prior to pouring it into the ear. I heard of a child the other day who had had raging earache due to the eruption of some back teeth, who fell asleep within five minutes of the *Plantago* being put into his ear, also *Plantago* may be taken internally and repeated every 3 to 4 hours.

Earache due to cold, coming on after exposure to cold winds, draughts, after infectious diseases such as measles, scarlet fever, whooping cough and tonsillitis is greatly eased by dropping in a drop or two of hot Mullein or *Verbascum* oil once or twice a day whenever the pain recurs. Internal medication may be needed as well. *Belladonna* is required when the face is highly flushed, burning red and hot and it will work miracles in relieving acute inflammations of the ear. *Ferrum phos.* has done the same in other cases, where the child had almost habitual earache returning at every exposure to draught ; it acted as a deterrent and prevented the earache, given in repeated doses whenever the pain returned. *Pulsatilla* is handy for cases after measles and whooping cough, after exposure to draughts and after getting wet feet ; such a child with earache is usually fretful and whiny. *Aconite* cures when the pain comes on within a short period of exposure to a cold wind, especially a north-east wind. The patient is anxious, restless and fearful during such an attack. *Chamomilla* will remove the pain rapidly if the patient is extremely irritable, in a rare paddy, hits and strikes, asks for things, throws them on the floor, one cheek red and hot, the other pale.

FROSTBITE

IN arctic weather, polar regions and on tops of high mountains, exposed parts of the body and the extremities, such as the nose, ears, toes and fingers may become frostbitten. First, all feeling is lost, then the parts become white and later congested and bluish in appearance. The individual may not be aware of it, as there is no sensation in the part affected, and the first warning he may get is the timely attention from a passer-by, who, seeing his plight will pick up some snow and rub the affected part; which will have the effect of stimulating the contracted blood vessels and by causing them to dilate will bring back the circulation to the frostbitten part.

The first rule in frostbite is mild friction with snow and later dry gentle heat until sensation and warmth are restored ; neglect of this precautionary measure may lead to gangrene of the frostbitten area. After the circulation has been restored, bring the patient into a warm room, give him hot drinks, hot soups, hot coffee, tea and, if severely exhausted, put him into a warm bed with the hot bottles properly wrapped round with blankets so that they do not touch the bare skin. *Ferrum phos.* may be needed as well, if the other measures are not sufficient.

Chilblains, which are a minor variety of frostbite, are best treated by local application of *Tamus communis* tincture ; the tincture is made from the berries of the Black Bryony which are steeped in gin and then used as a paint for chilblains. Should they break, apply *Calendula* lotion on top of *Calendula* ointment, and when it is healing, *Calendula* ointment by itself. Internally, *Agaricus, Pulsatilla, Sulphur* or *Hepar sulph.* may be necessary. Inflamed, intensely itching, purple chilblains which are worse from heat, worse in a warm room, worse in a hot bed, worse sitting in front of a fire, require *Pulsatilla.* Septic broken chilblains which itch and burn and are worse in the cold, require *Petroleum.* Chilblains of the feet, toes and hands which are worse in the cold and better in the warmth, need *Agaricus.* Suppurating chilblains which are very painful and tender to touch, need *Hepar sulph.* Where there is much burning and intense itching with dark - red inflammation which is covered with blisters, worse in the damp cold, *Rhus tox.* will cure ; itching purple and suppurating chilblains need *Sulphur.*

For prevention of chilblains, apply gentle rotary massage up the toes and up the fingers and hands at the beginning of the cold season. Lanoline, lambswool fat, rubbed into the skin in the manner described is almost infallible in preventing them. Calcium injections and Calcium medications are quite unnecessary in my opinion. Extra fat in the diet is necessary, extra butter, extra milk or extra pea-nut butter, or even cod-liver oil, if the person concerned can digest it. If extra fat and extra milk are taken, I do not think there is any need for vitamin medication, provided that local friction with animal fat, such as Lanoline, is not forgotten.

Whether the old gipsy remedy of washing the hands and feet covered in chilblains with the sufferer's own urine is always efficacious I am not prepared to say, but it has answered well in some cases. Desperate cases need desperate remedies, and when there is a shortage of fats in the diet and difficulty of supplies of ointment bases, my last suggestion may be worth a trial.

RUPTURE, HERNIA

A RUPTURE is a protrusion of the bowel through the muscular wall of the abdomen under the skin and may come on suddenly through over-exertion, over-lifting or heavy muscular work of any kind. The symptoms are sudden swelling and pain coming on after any heavy exertion. Mr. Carleton in his book, *Methods in Medicine and Surgery*, mentions several cases which have been cured and remained cured for many years after weekly doses of *Nux vomica* in a high potency. In some cases a truss has been necessary for a time while the remedy was doing its work.

In children, especially in fat, flabby babies with inguinal hernia—rupture of the groin—*Calcarea carb.* has been successful. Umbilical hernia in infants can usually be cured in a few weeks by approximating the sides of the abdomen and putting over it strips of adhesive plaster, two inches wide and long enough to go half round the body. The occasional exception can usually be cured with *Calcarea carb.* or *Nux vomica*. *Calcarea carb.* in a fat, phlegmatic infant, and *Nux vomica* for the lean kine.

POISONS

POISONS should be treated by elimination, neutralization with the chemical antidote, as well as attention to shock. Give an emetic, if there is no sign of burning of the lips and mouth : such as a tablespoonful of mustard powder in half a pint of luke-warm water or salt in a tumblerful of luke-warm water, repeating the emetic, until the patient vomits. If lips and mouth are burnt no emetic should be given but a neutralizing antidote will be necessary.

If the poison taken was an acid, give large quantities of an alkali, lime water or a tablespoonful of whitening or chalk or magnesia ; if the poison taken was an alkali, give vinegar or lemon juice, if available, diluted with equal parts water, drunk by the tumblerful. Carbolic acid and Lysol poisoning needs Epsom or Glauber's salts, dissolved in a tumblerful of milk or water for an antidote. For corrosive sublimate = perchloride of mercury, give white of egg mixed in water in large quantities, after which give an emetic. The treatment for Iodine poisoning is starch and water mixed or large quantities of thin cornflour or arrowroot which will turn the poisonous iodine chemically into a harmless iodide salt.

In Phosphorus poisoning, give Epsom or Glauber salts, one tablespoonful in a tumbler of water, no oil or fat should be given in any form. In alcoholic poisoning, the patient must be kept warm so as to prevent pneumonia as a result from exposure, the stomach may have to be washed out with warm water, using a stomach pump. Internally *Ledum* antidotes the effect of whisky ; and *Coffea* in potency is of great help for sobering up.

Shock must be treated in all cases of poisoning with rest, hot bottles and hot drinks as soon as consciousness returns ; medicinally *Aconite* may be given, if the patient is anxious, scared, restless and afraid, which happens, if he has taken the poison by accident. *Ignatia*, if he is hysterical and weepy. *Arnica*, if he feels bruised, sleepy and comatose. Some of the poisons can be antidoted by giving it in potency such as potentized *Phosphorus* for Phosphorus poisoning, or an *Arsenic* potency in Arsenic poisoning ; but attend to the elimination and chemical anti- doting first and foremost in cases of acute poisoning.

Snake bite should be treated by a local application to the wound of a solution of Permanganate of Potash and constriction of the arm or thigh between the wound and the heart, thus arresting circulation in the limbs, by tying braces or strips of clothing or making use of an improvised tourniquet round the limb. Keep the constriction in position for fifteen minutes, then relax for one minute, after which tighten up again. Strong coffee should be given, if the patient is conscious. If the snake venom is known, give it in the 30th potency such as *Naja* for a bite from the cobra ; *Lachesis* 30 for a bite from the South American Surukuku snake and so on. *Vipera* 12th potency in a bite from the British adder.

BOILS AND CARBUNCLES

BOILS and Carbuncles are extremely painful, unpleasant and unsightly things to combat. The treatments given are varied, usually protracted and uncertain in their results. Those unfortunate people who are afflicted with boils never seem able to cope with them successfully; they are pursued by them for months and years in some cases. In Homœopathy we have at least one if not more remedies which give brilliant results, and at the same time without needing the assistance of the surgeon and his scalpel. For nearly eight years at least I have scarcely ever used the knife to open a boil or even a carbuncle, but have relied in every case on *Tarentula cubensis*; and locally on the use of *Hypericum* tincture at a dilution of 1 in 25, in tepid or even cold applications renewed every 4 to 6 hours in acute cases, in addition to *Tarentula cubensis* internally 3 to 4 times daily. In a large number of cases, the carbuncle was absorbed, it just seemed to disappear without the patient showing any ill effects after it. In rare cases there was a recurrence of the carbuncle; it was quite exceptional for the patient to return for treatment for a second crop of boils or carbuncles. If he did, the same treatment used to suffice to clear him up in a few days. It was remarkable to see young lads with a history of ten to twelve to eighteen boils in the previous three to four months clear up within a week or less of large boils without any surgical interference, with the minimum of pain and with no recurrence except in the rarest of instances. Out of about sixty cases treated in the last eight years I can recall only three cases who suffered from more than one siege of their enemy after the application of this treatment : *Hypericum* externally and *Tarentula cubensis* internally.

There was a lad who came with an enormous carbuncle in his groin near the scrotum. He could neither sit, nor stand, nor walk upright, he came in bent over like an old man. A tepid *Hypericum* compress 3 times daily and *Tarentula cubensis* thrice a day eased him so much that when he was seen two days later, the swelling had disappeared and only a small hard patch was left behind. He had slept, he could eat again, and he walked in upright and smiling. It was completely healed in five days with no recurrence.

Another boy with a large carbuncle on the left side of his neck under the jaw, the size of a small hen's egg, a hard swelling with pitting on pressure, dusky red, almost purple in colour, it became larger and more prominent at first under treatment, fluctuating so that I was almost tempted to open it under Ethyl chloride, but my medical scalpel did not fail me at the last. It was absorbed completely without leaving a trace after twelve days' treatment, the boy's general health improving the whole time. There was a slight recurrence at the back of the neck during the next fortnight which only lasted two or three days, he looked well and flourishing at the end of it, thanks to *Tarentula cubensis* internally and *Hypericum* externally. " An outstanding case," as the Sister of the clinic remarked. " One of many," was my retort.

There are some other remedies noted down for boils and carbuncles, but so far I have never had to use them. *Tarentula cubensis* has filled the bill. *Arnica* may be required when a case is seen which presents crops of septic pimples, a few doses will suffice to remove them.

SEPTIC CONDITIONS, WHITLOWS, ETC.

THE local treatment for these septic conditions is *Hypericum* dressings which can be assisted greatly by internal medication. I was scratched by the side of the thumbnail near the quick by a cat, within an hour or two it began to throb and swell, it felt hot and looked purple. I developed a temperature and could not settle down to anything, wandering restlessly about the room. I felt thirsty, but could not drink much at a time, had a desire for hot tea. On these symptoms I took *Arsenic* and went to sleep within a few minutes and slept all night. *Hypericum* dressings were changed frequently, pus began to flow freely from the sinus which extended right down to the bone. I repeated *Arsenic* whenever the finger did not feel so comfortable. If I had been able to rest the finger it would have been well in two or three days, but due to constantly using it the healing was delayed for a fortnight ; but I had no pain after the first three hours, when it was removed by *Arsenic*.

A young girl came to the Centre with a septic tenosynovitis—inflammation of the flexor tendon of the middle-finger—due to a neglected cut sustained ten days previously. The finger was badly swollen, deep purple, and excruciatingly tender. *Hypericum* was applied and *Hypericum* given internally ; when seen the next day there was no change in the condition. I made a superficial opening along the course of the tendon, where the pus was pointing, under a local anæsthetic, to let it out. A cold *Hypericum* dressing was applied and the girl remarked with a pleased thrill in her voice, " Oh, it's cold, how nice." On this : relief from cold application, she was given *Pulsatilla*, repeated twice daily. Two days later the finger was almost entirely healed from the bottom of the wound up. I have never seen such a rapid change in a septic tendon in all the years of my professional life. She was discharged five days after with a perfectly sound finger which was straight, with a perfect range of movements—there was no stiffness whatsoever and no massage was needed after it.

SUFFOCATION DUE TO CARBON MONOXIDE—COAL GAS POISONING

CARBON monoxide poisoning is not uncommon these days when so many people possess motor cars. It is the gas which is generated in petrol engines and is the cause of suffocation in badly ventilated garages, when the car is left running and the gas escaping from the exhaust pipe fills an enclosed space. The gas is odourless and colourless and cannot be detected therefore. This is also the gas given off from defective hot-water geysers in bathrooms, the defect often leading to fatalities. If gas is suspected in a room where there is an unconscious person a gas mask should be worn on entering. The windows should be opened wide in order to allow free circulation of air to disperse the gas. The patient should be removed as quickly as possible and artificial respiration should be performed immediately, and *Carbo veg.* in granules given in repeated doses every ten minutes, dry on the tongue until consciousness returns, when the doses can be spaced at longer intervals. In slight cases of gas poisoning, *Bryonia* will be effectual. Remember that in coal gas poisoning the face of the patient looks pinker than normal and he thus appears to be in the best of health ; therefore do not be misled by it.

SOME MEDICAL EMERGENCIES

LET us consider a few minor medical emergencies such as food poisoning, which consists in a sudden attack of vomiting and diarrhœa and is usually called Ptomaine poisoning ; a sudden attack which comes on with a feeling of nausea, vomiting of everything that is taken, great weakness, a dry mouth and fearful anxiety and restlessness, everything burns that enters the stomach or comes up. Sips of warm water may be comforting. Heat applied externally is also pleasant ; dysenteric symptoms may be present with straining and burning at the anus. The cause of this condition can often be traced back to eating spoilt and decayed animal matter, bad sausages, bad meat, which may have been suitably disguised with condiments by the restaurant keeper ; drinking of ice cold water or eating ice cream may bring on similar symptoms. *Arsenic* repeated, whenever the symptoms recur, will cure rapidly.

A *Bryonia* case is one where the patient has been over-eating. He suffers violent pain in the abdomen, severe vomiting, he can keep nothing down, and even though he is thirsty, cold water will return as soon as it enters the stomach ; he is worse for motion, lies perfectly still, with the limbs flexed, knees drawn up, the pains in his stomach are relieved by hot applications, the nausea and vomiting comes on whenever he raises his head and tries to sit up. These symptoms may be due, as I say, to an excess of food or follow after rich food, after cabbage, old cheese, new bread, ice cream and may even indicate the first stage of appendicitis and will cure appendicitis, *if the symptoms here mentioned are present*. Repeat *Bryonia* whenever there is a recurrence of the trouble—pain, vomiting, etc.

Pulsatilla may be necessary and will cure some cases of acute gastric disturbance, coming on after eating pork or pastry, or bad fish, bad meat, ice cream. The symptoms are nausea, bloating of the stomach, colicky pains, belching up of rancid food, slimy mouth, bad taste in the mouth, dryness of the mouth, but he is practically never thirsty, restlessness with improvement from walking about slowly, cannot lie still with gastric and bowel symptoms, likes fresh air and the windows open.

Carbo veg. for cases of acute indigestion after eating pork, rich food, spoiled fish, bad meat, excess of fat or rancid fat, the principal symptoms are accumulation of wind, distension of the stomach, everything turns to wind, is always belching, full of anxiety and restlessness with distension mainly on lying down at night, worse on lying down and is relieved by sitting up and by loud eructations.

China indigestion and colic comes on after excess of fruit, after eating cabbage, raw vegetables, drinking too much tea and eating sour things such as pickles, bad fish and flatulent food, etc. Distended, bloated stomach with constant belching without any relief, different from *Carbo veg.*—light touch makes pain and indigestion worse, while firm pressure relieves. Diarrhœa after eating, rumbling in the abdomen and expelling of quantities of wind from the bowels, yellow, painless stools.

Saccharine poisoning was a comparatively common complaint in the days of sugar rationing, when the sweet-tooth felt hardly done by and tried to supplement his sugar ration with Saccharine. Many cases of poisoning are stigmatized gastric influenza, when the trouble is entirely due to the sensitivity of the patient to Saccharine. The symptoms may come on within an hour or two after eating some kinds of sweets, sweet cakes, or putting Saccharine in tea or coffee. The victim may not always know that he has had Saccharine. The symptoms are those of extreme cold, chilly feeling and shivering down the back to the legs, extreme collapse, violent thirst which makes the shivering worse, vomiting of bile at the end of the chilly period, then feelings of heat come on, intense heat with excessive aching deep in the bones of the back and limbs, so intense that there is constant movement and restlessness. The aching is so intense that the patient tells you that he feels the bones will break ; there is no sweating. *Eupatorium perfoliatum* will relieve quickly in such cases ; doses to be repeated whenever pains or sickness recur.

The common bilious attack is usually rapidly put right by a few doses of *Nux vomica* if the symptoms are as follows : an attack comes on after exposure to a cold dry wind or draught. The biliousness is due to the partaking of too rich food, drinking too many sherries and bitters, followed by strong coffee ; this brings on heaviness and weight in the stomach and chest a couple of hours after a meal, and a general sensation of cold, " livery " feeling, nausea, sometimes retching, jaundiced eyes and skin, constipation, piles, all associated with great irritability and snappiness. Such a person lives on laxatives and tonics which make the last state worse than the first. He becomes more and more dyspeptic and livery and more and more difficult to live with. Given *Nux vomica* in repeated doses, he will become amiable, get rid of his biliousness and will be generally improved in health and temper.

There are certain people who inflict this earth who believe that small doses of Glauber's salts taken in their morning tea is a cure-all for rheumatism and constipation and will give them that feeling of being able to jump over the moon, while as a matter of fact it produces the very things they are trying to eliminate. The constant draining of the liver weakens the constitution and produces slow digestion, nausea with squeamishness after starchy food, vomiting of bile with colic, pain in the abdomen, fullness and rumbling and gurgling, diarrhœa alternating with constipation, morning diarrhœa, great sensitiveness to damp weather, violent headaches and pains in the joints and sciatica. Stop the daily morning dose and take a few doses of potentized *Natrum sulph.* for a short time. The biliousness and livery feeling will disappear and the feeling of joy and happiness will be the reward.

HEADACHES

The first thing that people will have to forswear in order to get cured of headaches is the constant doping with Aspirin. It is a bad habit and leads to other troubles. More and more headaches, heart weakness, nervous depression, even the very teeth give up the ghost and shed their enamel after over-dosing with Aspirin, which inevitably leads to premature loss of teeth and the gaining of dentures, to say nothing of a more or less chronic state of indigestion and an inability to enjoy life. What then do I suggest instead of Aspirin which has become such a habit during the last few decades ? The chronic sufferer from headaches should first reconsider his mode of life, late hours, drinking too many cocktails, rushing about with no time for rest and no leisure for thought, dancing through half the night in vitiated air, going to work after too little sleep, working for long hours under the glare of badly placed lighting, insufficient food or the wrong kind, buns and too much tea ; all these are some of the causes for headaches and could and should be avoided. Aspirin does take a headache away, I admit, but it adds more trouble to the already overdrawn exchequer on the Bank of Health. Cut off the causes, some of which are given here, and there will be less incitement to take such a harmful habit-forming drug as Aspirin. Follow ordinary simple health rules : have as much fresh air as you can after the hours spent in office or factory, walk to and from work whenever possible, drink less strong tea and coffee, eat as much fruit and raw vegetables, either chopped or grated, as you can, drink vegetable water and have simple food properly cooked at regular intervals as far as possible ; go to bed at reasonable hours to get your full quota of sleep. Find out the cause of the headache, if it is not due to any of these causes, take yourself to task and try to remember what might have brought it on. If due to indigestion, constipation or too many laxatives, take *Nux vomica*, night and morning for a few days until the headache improves and finally disappears.

If the headache is due to over eating, a full stomach, too much fat, too much ice cream, *Pulsatilla* will help, taken hourly or 2 hourly while the headache is severe and leaving off as soon as the headache is gone.

If the headache is brought on by sorrow, emotion, grief or worry, *Ignatia* will usually help, taken in the same way as suggested for *Pulsatilla*.

If headaches come on after a fall or injury or concussion, take *Arnica* hourly, until improvement sets in.

If the headache is the result of too long an exposure to the sun, *Belladonna* will relieve quickly red, flushed face, throbbing in the head, throbbing in the arteries, and a great rush of blood to the head. *Glonoine* may be necessary in some cases as this kind of headache is usually a mild type of sunstroke ; it is usually worse from lying down, with fullness and pain at the back of the head and neck. Relief is obtained by sitting up and pressing the back of the head.

Migraine and sick headaches are periodical headaches, coming on every eight days or every fortnight or less often ; these are relieved frequently by *Iris*. This headache begins with a blur before the eyes, with a throbbing and shooting in the forehead with nausea and vomiting of sour food, profuse flow of saliva, and severe burning in the anus with straining and bearing down, crampy pains everywhere.

Headaches in children from anticipation and excitement so that when the promised treat is due, the child is laid low with violent headache and sickness, can usually be rapidly cured with either *Arsenic* or *Gelsemium*. The *Arsenic* child is excitable and restless and gets these violent attacks of headaches and vomiting when he brings up everything, even the smallest quantity of water. A few doses of *Arsenic*, while the sickness and headache lasts will soon remove this bugbear. Before the next party is due give the child 3 doses of *Arsenic* in 24 hours. This will quieten the restless excitability so that he can look forward to and enjoy the treat.

Gelsemium is for the child who suffers from nerves, due to anticipation, fear and effects of sudden surprises which make him weak, faint and exhausted, violent hammering pains in the head. He has to go to bed, lying there dazed and almost too weak to move. Frequently there are palpitations and diarrhœa. *Gelsemium* will conquer all this and turn him into a quieter, less fearful, less nervous individual.

COLDS AND CHILLS

Colds and chills often need emergency treatment so as to prevent serious trouble developing. A stitch in time . . .

In the southern counties of England personal experience has taught me that in the majority of cases *Arsenicum* taken, as soon as the first signs of a cold show themselves, in $\frac{1}{2}$ hourly doses (4 to 6 as a rule) will abort it, unless the chill is due to standing in a howling north-easterly gale on a cold, draughty railway platform or while waiting for infrequent buses, then *Aconite*, taken in the same manner as suggested for *Arsenic*, usually will keep the enemy at bay.

Allium cepa, our friend, the common onion, will do wonders in certain colds and nasal catarrhs where the nasal discharge is acrid and burning in character, the freely flowing watery discharge from the eyes is bland and painless, the patient feels worse in a warm room and worse in the evening, when the exciting cause of the cold is exposure to cold north-east winds. It should be taken as before, ½ hourly until signs of a cold are disappearing.

Nux vomica colds and chills come on after exposure to cold winds, with fluent coryza in the morning and during the daytime with stoppage of flow at night ; the free flowing discharge of mucus from one nostril which seems obstructed by dry catarrh, feelings of chilliness on the slightest movement, the patient cannot get warm, although sitting over the fire or even when well covered with warm bedclothing. There is also extreme irritability, snappiness, a " nothing is right " feeling.

These are some of the more common cold remedies, though others may be required.

ON POTENCIES

THROUGHOUT these pages I have repeatedly mentioned many remedies by name without qualifying them as to dose and potencies. Let me explain to those who have little or no knowledge of the art and science of Homœopathy, that potency means power, and is the energy or activity latent in each drug, brought out by the special mode of preparation. The nearest approach to a fuller understanding of what is meant by potentizing is the colloidal action of substances in orthodox medicine. Colloids are suspensions of exceedingly small globules of solute in the solvent and include thus amorphous, gelatinous, glue-like forms. There is no actual physical solution brought about in potentizing a drug, but a breaking-up into minute particles, each of which retains the full activity and powers of the drug.

Potentizing practically and briefly explained, means the dilution of a drug by adding and mixing a specific minute quantity with a certain specific quantity of a diluent vehicle which is non-medicinal, such as water or alcohol. This mixture of drug and diluent is then vigorously shaken or percussed in a liquid medium ; in the case of a solid it is rubbed down or triturated with a definite quantity of sugar of milk as the inert diluent. This vigorous shaking or grinding breaks down the walls of the cells making up the drug and frees the dynamic energy. The most important part of the process of potentizing is not the dilution of the drug but the active vibrations set up by the shaking, while the dilutions are carried out at a definite arithmetical ratio. The first centesimal potency is made from the original tincture and stands for one in a hundred dilution. The second centesimal potency is made from the first, by taking one drop of the first to ninety-nine drops of the diluent and shaking vigorously, so with each rising potency, one drop of the previous is diluted with the same quantity of diluting vehicle and shaken vigorously. This process can be carried on almost indefinitely, providing at each step it is well shaken and thoroughly mixed, thus releasing the latent and hidden radioactivity—if we may call it this—of a drug. The lower potencies are more closely related to the chemical and physiological action of a drug, while the higher potencies produce effects that are entirely dynamic and often of far reaching and unsuspected depth and extent ; in length of time of action, a dose of a high potency shakes up the entire vital energy or force of a human being and should not be lightly used, except by somebody with the deepest understanding and knowledge of the action of each drug and the total drug picture as produced on a healthy person during the process of finding out its complete symptomatology. The lower potencies are safer for use by doctors, inexperienced as yet in Homœopathy, as well as for the lay persons. The higher potency therefore should be left to the discretion of the experienced homœopathic physician to order when he considers it necessary. By a lower potency I include those up to the third or even the sixth potency which can be handled with comparative safety by the mere tyro.

The *repetition* of the dose depends entirely on the severity or virulence of the disease process. The more active or virulent the disease, the more frequently must the medicine be repeated ; in such an acute disease condition, such as severe pain, troublesome cough, diarrhœa, vomiting, etc., the medicine may have to be repeated as often as every 10 to 15 minutes, until the patient gets relief from the pain, or the vomiting ceases or the diarrhœa stops, or the cough gets easier or he sinks into a natural sleep. All these various reactions indicate that the medicine is doing its work, and while the patient sleeps and while the improvement continues, there is no necessity to repeat the medicine.

The first grand rule of repetition of homœopathic medicine is : *let each dose act to its fullest capacity, do not repeat or give a second dose unless there is a recurrence of cough, pain, sickness, diarrhœa or when the patient awakes.* This may be, as I have said, after a few minutes in very acute conditions, or in less acute conditions it may not happen for two, three, four hours or longer. The patient who has been given the correct homœopathic medicine—given

according to the Law of Similars, that is " Like Cures Like "—
will definitely know without having to be told whether the
medicine is doing him good ; he will have a sense of well being
which he will never experience after a dose of Aspirin or any
other palliative medicine.   They may remove the pain for the
time being, but they do not *heal* and restore the patient's vital
energy ; hence there is no feeling of well being.

Let me once more emphasize, do not repeat the medicine
or the dose until there is a recurrence of troublesome symptoms.
In the lower potencies there is no necessity for such accurate
and detailed diagnosis of a drug, as many drugs resemble each
other in their symptoms and frequently do one another's work
and carry on the healing process, although the time factor may
be longer.   For example : the most similar remedy for a certain
disease may be recognized as *Bryonia*, by the experienced and
knowledgeable homœopathic physician in an acute condition,
this will cure pneumonia, let us say, in two to three days, as has
happened frequently, while the less experienced doctor or lay
person may give *Aconite* and then *Belladonna* and then *Ferrum
phos.* and so on, and gradually pneumonia will be conquered in
eight or nine days, instead of in two to three days by the " homœopathic most similar " remedy.

Or whooping cough may be absolutely eradicated in 24
to 48 hours by one dose of a high potency of *Drosera* which
again is a well-known fact to the homœopathic physician,
while the less knowledgeable doctor or lay person by giving his
Aconite and *Ipecac.* and *Antimonium tart.* will achieve the same
result eventually in three to four weeks.   This is where the art
of the experienced physician with his knowledge of the individual
drugs comes in.

But the higher potencies even though they may cure dramatic-
ally with one or two doses of the correct drug are like a two-
edged sword in the hands of an inexperienced prescriber who
first of all may *not* know his drugs so well and secondly does not
realize the depth of the disturbance of the vital reaction it calls
forth, and that a second or a third dose should never be given
until the action of each dose is fully expended.   If the doses are
repeated too quickly a serious collapse may ensue, the symptoms
may return with renewed vigour and the alarmed prescriber may

then go to another drug and set up further complications. A vast knowledge of homœopathic philosophy and a deep understanding of action and reaction are necessary, before a prescriber should venture into the realms of dynamic infinitesimal doses. Forsooth the saying is true: " a little knowledge is a dangerous thing."

It may be necessary to change prescriptions in acute cases if there is no response to a remedy, that is, if there is no change in the condition. Wait at least six hours before reconsidering a case in an acute state, meanwhile meticulously collecting all the symptoms from the patient, the patient's relatives and/or the nurse. This means careful training of all the people who have to do with looking after a sick person. It is astounding how few people know what to look for in recording a patient's symptoms and reactions and often a prescriber must stay at the bedside for a considerable time or see a patient repeatedly, before he is able to find the correct, indicated remedy. It is not so difficult of course in such cases as I have described in this booklet, as accidents and injuries require more or less the same specific remedies.

Let me repeat that the medicines to which reference has been made, should be used in the lower potencies only by the first-aider or in the home. The 3 or 6 potencies work very well and no potency above the sixth centesimal should be used until the prescriber is sure of his ground and knows the different remedies in relationship with the various similar and contrasting drugs extremely well. Each medicine should be *repeated only when there is a return of troublesome symptoms* ; in acute conditions the medicines should not be continued for an indefinite period, but the medication should cease twenty-four hours after the temperature is down or the cough has ceased, or the pain gone ; in fact when the patient feels well. On the other hand, the lowest potencies such as mother tincture or the 1*x* potency of poisonous drugs, such as *Aconite* or *Nux vomica* should never be ordered, they are too near the danger line, the physiologically or chemically toxic effects.

The full knowledge of correct potencies is a study of a lifetime, wide experience and deep research. It is better to start using low potencies until with increased knowledge and wisdom the higher potencies may be used with the greatest caution. All potencies work, from the first to the hundred-thousandth, but the physician must remember that there is a best (an optimum) potency for every individual. *Weak and elderly individuals require low potencies and young and active people can be given medium and higher potencies ; but for the newcomer in Homœopathy the lower potencies are always the best to use.*

The correctly indicated remedy given according to the law of similars works in any potency, including the lower ones, so if a doctor or a lay person prefers to use the 3rd decimal (3*x*) potencies or the 6*x* (sixth decimal) there is no reason why he should not obtain good results provided he stops while the *improvement is maintained.*

A few more words must be added regarding the preparation, handling and storage of these remedies. In the first instance they should be obtained direct from homœopathic chemists at any rate until such times as the general pharmacists learn to appreciate the value of homœopathic drugs and the extreme care which is needed in handling and storing them ; and that one drug will not necessarily replace another, even though it is prescribed in quantities of one millionth or smaller. As regards handling and storing, the remedies should be kept in a cool, dry and preferably dark place, in special cupboards or chests, where no other strong-smelling lotions, liniments, such as menthol, camphor, peppermint essences, scents, etc., are kept as these will antidote the action of the delicately poised homœopathic remedies and make them inert. If carefully stored and handled, these remedies will not deteriorate but keep their power for many years except perhaps in the case of the strong mother tinctures which act better when recently made from fresh material. As far as possible, each dose should be given to the patient direct without undue handling, by this I mean that the remedy should be taken from the bottle or container on to a piece of paper and the fingers or paper should not be put into the bottle in order to remove a pilule or dose.

While taking homœopathic remedies the patient should be careful to refrain from taking other medicines, sleeping draughts, etc. He should not rub strong smelling antiseptics or liniments into the skin, he should not use antiseptic toothpastes and mouth washes, but rely on soap and water, or charcoal for cleansing the teeth and a weak *Calendula* solution for a mouth wash.

Certain articles of diet are also forbidden, such as strong coffee, condiments, heavy spices ; peppermint sweets and cough lozenges should not be taken, if the maximum benefit from the drugs is to be obtained.

SUGGESTED INTERNAL REMEDIES
FOR THE FIRST-AID BOX

Aconite—chills, effect of fear, shock, fright.

Arnica—bruises, shock, contusions, injuries.

Arsenic—food poisoning, colds.

Belladonna—mild sunstroke, headache, earache.

Bryonia—biliousness, liverishness, colds, chills, influenza.

Calendula—cuts and incised wounds.

Carbo veg.—indigestion, flatulence.

Causticum—burns.

Cantharides—burns.

Chamomilla—in teething children, in acute earache.

China—indigestion, diarrhœa.

Coffea—wakefulness, fainting from shock.

Eupatorium—saccharine poisoning and influenza.

Ferrum phos.—earache.

Gelsemium—headache, chills, influenza.

Glonoine—headaches due to heatstroke.

Hamamelis—bleeding from veins.

Hepar sulph.—septic wounds, extremely painful and tender to touch.

Hypericum—lacerations, crushing, pains in the coccyx after childbirth, or falls on the coccyx.

Ignatia—nerves, grief, shock and fainting.

Ipecacuanha—faintness with nausea, hæmorrhages.

Iris—Migraine headaches.

Ledum—punctured wounds, black eye.

Nux vomica—biliousness.

Opium—headaches.

Phosphorus—hæmorrhage, teeth extraction.

Pulsatilla—indigestion after fat, getting feet wet, colds.

Rhus tox.—sprains and strains.

Ruta—bruised periosteum, bones.

Silica—sepsis.

Symphytum—bones after fractures.
Tarentula cubensis 6—boils, carbuncles.
Urtica urens—burns.
Vipera 12—nose-bleeding.

TINCTURES FOR EXTERNAL USE

Arnica.
Calendula.
Hypericum.
Plantago—in toothache for application to gums and ears.
Tamus communis—for chilblains.

OINTMENTS FOR APPLICATION

Arnica.
Calendula.
Hypericum.
Ruta.
Symphytum.

INDEX